EXECUTIVE SUMMARY

PURPOSE

This inspection surveyed junior and senior high school (7th through 12 grade) students to determine how they obtain, view, and consume alcohol.

BACKGROUND

In response to public health concerns and the adverse health consequences of alcohol abuse, Surgeon General Antonia Novello requested that the Office of Inspector General (OIG) survey youth to determine their views and practices regarding alcohol use. These concerns mirror one of Department of Health and Human Services (HHS) Secretary Louis Sullivan's goals which is to reduce the prevalence of alcohol problems among children and youth. The Surgeon General is particularly concerned about the drinking habits of youth, especially the nation's 20.7 million 7th through 12th graders. This report is one in a series prepared by the OIG related to youth and alcohol. It describes survey findings relating to youth perceptions, knowledge, opinions, and drinking habits and is based on structured interviews conducted with a random national sample of junior and senior high school students.

FINDINGS

▶ *Fifty-one percent of junior and senior high school students have had at least one drink within the past year and 8 million students drink weekly.*

▶ *Junior and senior high school students drink 35 percent of all wine coolers sold in the United States and 1.1 billion cans of beer each year.*

▶ *More than 5 million students have binged; 3 million within the last month; 454,000 binge at least once a week.*

▶ *More than 3 million students drink alone, more than 4 million drink when they are upset, and less than 3 million drink because they are bored.*

▶ *Students lack essential knowledge about alcohol and its effects.*

▶ *Nine million students get their information about alcohol from unreliable sources.*

▶ *Seven million students are able to walk into a store and buy alcohol.*

▶ *Students accept rides from friends who have been drinking.*

▸ *Parents, friends, and alcoholic beverage advertisements influence students' attitudes about alcohol.*

RECOMMENDATIONS

▸ *The Surgeon General should consult with public and private agencies to develop, improve, and promote educational programs which would increase student awareness of alcoholic beverages and their effects.*

▸ *The Surgeon General should collaborate with the appropriate public and private agencies to reduce the appeal of alcoholic beverage advertising to youth.*

▸ *The Surgeon General should emphasize the need for law enforcement and State alcoholic beverage control agencies to prevent youth from illegally purchasing alcohol.*

TABLE OF CONTENTS

iv

INTRODUCTION

PURPOSE

This inspection surveyed junior and senior high (7th through 12th grade) students to determine how they obtain, view, and consume alcohol.

BACKGROUND

In response to public health concerns and the adverse health consequences of alcohol abuse, Surgeon General Antonia Novello requested that the Office of Inspector General (OIG) survey youth to determine their views and practices regarding alcohol use. These concerns mirror one of Department of Health and Human Services (HHS) Secretary Louis Sullivan's goals which is to reduce the prevalence of alcohol problems among children and youth. The Surgeon General is particularly concerned about the drinking habits of youth, especially the nation's 20.7 million 7th through 12th graders. This report is one in a series prepared by the OIG related to youth and alcohol. It describes survey findings concerning youth perceptions, knowledge, opinions, and drinking habits.

Youth Consumption and Beliefs About Alcohol

According to the U.S. Department of Education, 20.7 million students attend 7th through 12th grade. Previous national surveys have disclosed that most adolescents have tried alcohol and that many drink frequently. Among high school seniors in the class of 1990, 89.5 percent had used alcohol at least once, and 32.2 percent had experienced a "binge" of 5 or more drinks in a row within the past 2 weeks.[1] While recent surveys of high school students indicate an overall drop in drug use, alcohol use continues at a high rate.

According to another survey, adolescents have started drinking at earlier ages since 1978.[2] Although youth begin using alcohol at earlier ages, their information regarding its contents and effects may be faulty. A recent survey of 4th, 5th, and 6th graders found that only 21 percent consider wine coolers a drug, while 50 percent believe beer, wine, and liquor are drugs.[3]

---

[1]University of Michigan, Institute for Social Research, "Monitoring the Future: A Continuing Study of the Lifestyles and Values of Youth," January 1991.

[2]National Clearinghouse on Alcohol and Drug Issues (NCADI), "Alcohol and Youth," NCADI Alcohol Topics Fact Sheet, January 1987, p. 1.

[3]National Families in Action, "Wine Coolers Becoming Gateway Drug," Drug Abuse Update, no. 28, March 1989, p. 12.

Youth obtain alcohol from a variety of social and commercial sources. Although the minimum age to buy alcohol in all States is 21, studies show that youth are frequently able to obtain alcohol with little or no problem. While youth frequently find alcohol at parties without parental supervision and at friends' homes, they also obtain alcohol from retail outlets in a variety of ways. Youth may (1) have an older friend purchase alcohol, (2) buy from stores that are known to sell to minors, and/or (3) solicit a stranger to purchase alcohol.[4] In some areas, youth may simply purchase alcohol without being challenged by the vendor. According to a recent study, underage males were able to buy beer in 97 of 100 District of Columbia stores.[5]

METHODOLOGY

To establish the universe of 7th through 12th grade students, we compiled data on all secondary (junior and senior high schools), kindergarten through 8th grade (K-8), and kindergarten through 12th grade (K-12) schools in the United States. We weighted the States based upon the total number of schools. The eight randomly selected States were: California, Colorado, Florida, Illinois, Louisiana, New York, Ohio, and Pennsylvania. We obtained data on all target schools in the eight States from the U.S. Department of Education. After weighting each county in each State by the number of students, we randomly selected two counties in each State. We randomly selected two schools from each county list, without weighting, for a total sample of 32 schools.

During March and April 1991, we conducted structured interviews with a random national sample of 956 students in the 7th through 12th grades. We asked all students about their opinions and knowledge of alcohol. We asked about the personal experiences of students who had drunk at least one full alcoholic beverage in the past year. Throughout this report, we refer to these students as "students who drink." Of the students who never drank alcohol or had not had a drink during the past year, we asked about their perceptions and observations of their classmates who drink. We refer to these students as "non-drinkers." Appendix A contains a full description of the sample selection and methodology.

---

[4]Friedner D. Wittman, Ph.D., J.W. Grube, and P. Shane, "Survey of Alcohol and Other Drug Experiences Among Castro Valley High School Students in 1987 and 1990," September 1, 1990, p. 2.

[5]Christine Russell, "It's Easy for Underage Men to Buy Beer in the District," Washington Post Health, March 19, 1991, p. 5.

FINDINGS

STATISTICAL HIGHLIGHTS: WHO DRINKS?

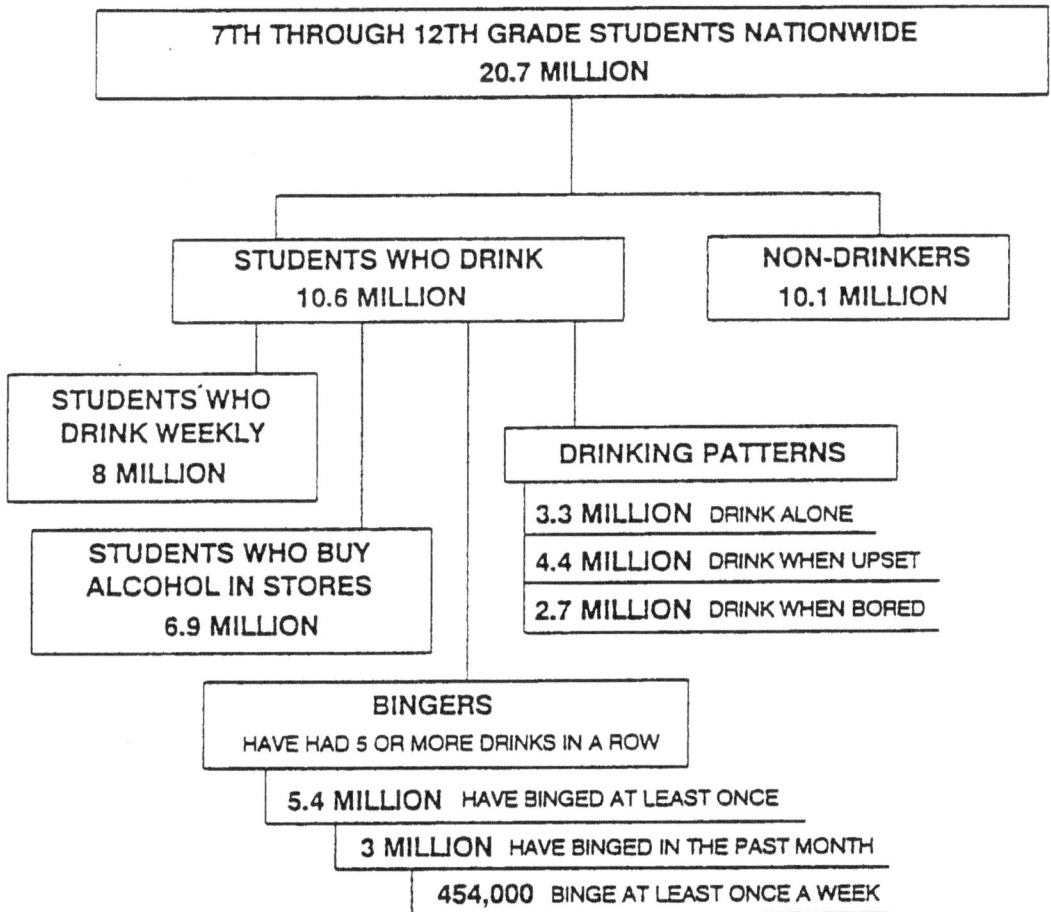

FIFTY-ONE PERCENT OF JUNIOR AND SENIOR HIGH SCHOOL STUDENTS HAVE HAD AT LEAST ONE DRINK WITHIN THE PAST YEAR.

According to our survey, 68 percent of all students have drunk alcohol at least once, and 51.2 percent (10.6 million) have had at least one drink within the past year. The average student who drinks is 16 years old and in the 10th grade. Of the students who drink, 53.8 percent are male, and 46.2 percent are female. See appendix B for gender and school grade breakdowns.

We found that students were 13 years old when they took their first drink. This is close to other national surveys that report 12.3 years as an average age.[6]

THE MAJORITY OF STUDENTS HAVE THEIR FIRST DRINK IN THEIR EARLY TEENS

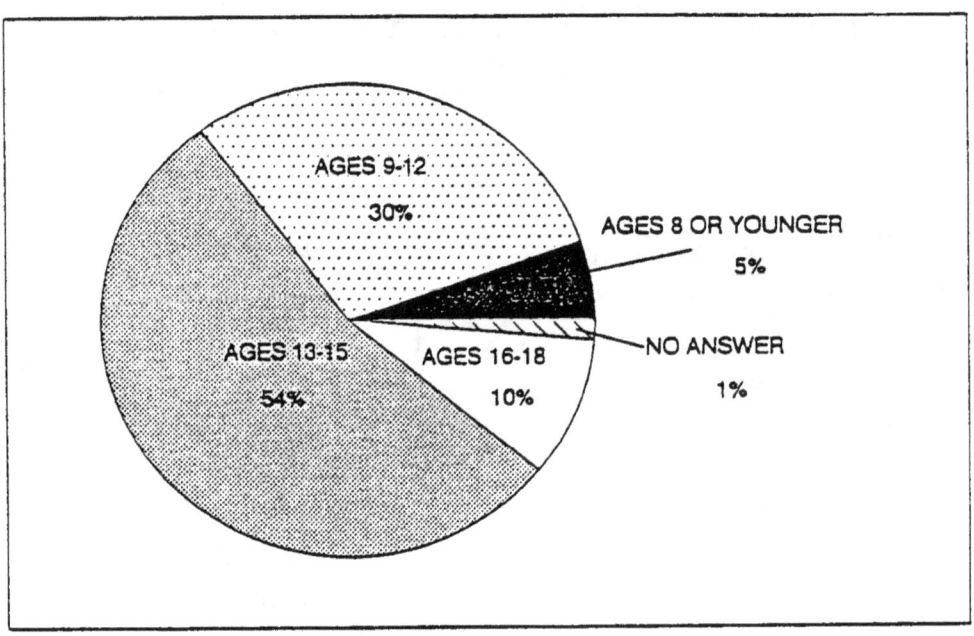

We found that eight million, or 38.6 percent of all students, drink weekly. Three million students reported that they do not usually drink each week.

JUNIOR AND SENIOR HIGH SCHOOL STUDENTS DRINK 35 PERCENT OF ALL WINE COOLERS SOLD IN THE UNITED STATES AND 1.1 BILLION CANS OF BEER EACH YEAR.

We asked students about four types of alcoholic beverages--beer (including all malt beverages), wine coolers, wine, and liquor (including mixed drinks that contain alcohol such as rum or vodka). Some students drink more than one type of alcoholic beverage. We project that:

▶ 9.2 million students have drunk beer. Of this group, 6 million drink between 0.12 and 33 beers weekly. In some schools, students mentioned that they

---

[6]U.S. Department of Health and Human Services, PHS-ADAMHA-OSAP, "Alcohol Use Among Children and Adolescents," Statistical Bulletin, October--December 1987, p. 2.

---

drink 40-ounce bottles of malt liquor instead of 12-ounce cans or bottles of beer.

► 8.9 million students have drunk wine coolers. Of this group, 4 million drink between 0.16 and 12 wine coolers weekly.

► 6.2 million students have drunk wine. Of this group, 1.4 million drink between 0.25 and 24 glasses of wine weekly.

► 7.2 million students have drunk liquor. Of this group, 3.6 million drink between 0.25 and 24 drinks weekly.

The average weekly consumption for each alcoholic beverage type is shown below.

WHILE WINE COOLERS ARE THE "DRINK OF CHOICE," STUDENTS DRINK MORE BEER

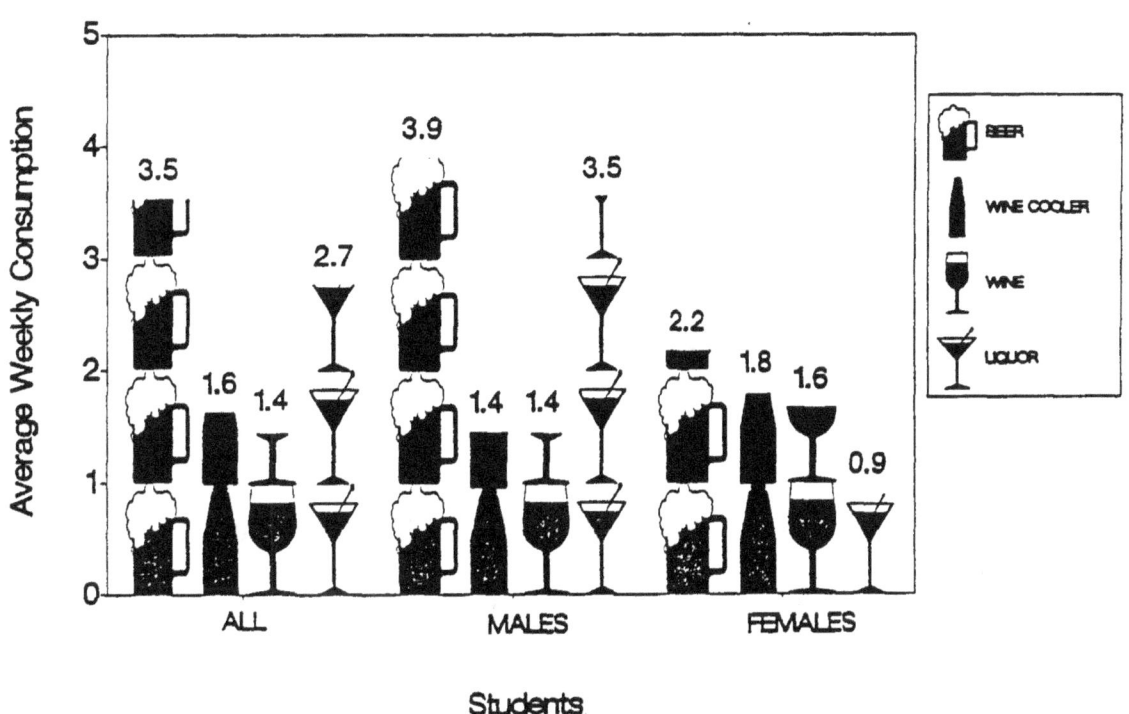

Wine coolers are the students' "drink of choice."

When asked about their favorite alcoholic drink, 42.1 percent of students who drink chose wine coolers. This translates to 4.5 million students who drink nationally. In addition, 51 percent of all students say that wine coolers are the favorite drink among their friends and classmates. Students choose wine coolers because they taste good, are fruity, do not have a strong taste of alcohol, and they think wine coolers do not contain much alcohol.

Junior and senior high school students drink 35 percent of all wine coolers sold in the United States.

According to estimated sales figures[7], 88.8 million gallons of wine coolers were sold in the United States in 1989. Based on an average consumption of 6.4 million bottles weekly (12-ounce size), we estimate that students drink 31.2 million gallons of wine coolers annually. By projecting the total volume of wine coolers students reported drinking, we estimate that students drink 35 percent of the wine coolers sold in this country.

Junior and senior high school students drink 1.1 billion beers each year.

Students drink less than 2 percent of the 62 billion bottles and cans[8] of beer consumed annually in the United States. While this percentage appears small, it is staggering when one considers that minors illegally consume more than a billion beers each year.

Students who chose beer as their favorite alcoholic beverage said it tastes good, is easy to get, is cheap, and does not get you drunk as fast as other alcoholic beverages. Several students said that beer is always around or available at parties.

MORE THAN 5 MILLION STUDENTS HAVE BINGED; 3 MILLION WITHIN THE LAST MONTH; 454,000 BINGE AT LEAST ONCE A WEEK.

Researchers define a "binge" as drinking five or more drinks in a row. Our projections show that 5.4 million students have "binged" at least once. Almost 55 percent of these had binged at least once in the month before the survey. For this group, the number of binges ranged from 1 to 20 per month.

The demographics for students who binge mirror the demographics for all students who drink. Fifty-nine percent are male; 41 percent female. The average binger is a 16-year-old male in the 10th grade. He was 12 years old when he took his first drink, slightly less than the average 13 years for all students who drink. He consumes six drinks each week.

---

[7]The Wine Institute, Table of Commercially Produced Wine Entering Distribution Channels in the United States, by Areas Where Produced, 1985--1989.

[8]1989 data, State reports compiled by Beer Institute and U.S. Department of Commerce, Bureau of Census.

There is a smaller group of students who binge almost every week--454,000 students average 15 drinks weekly. Their average age is 16.6 years, and they are in the 11th grade. Eighty-seven percent are males, and 13 percent are females.

BINGERS DRINK MORE BEER THAN OTHER ALCOHOLIC BEVERAGES

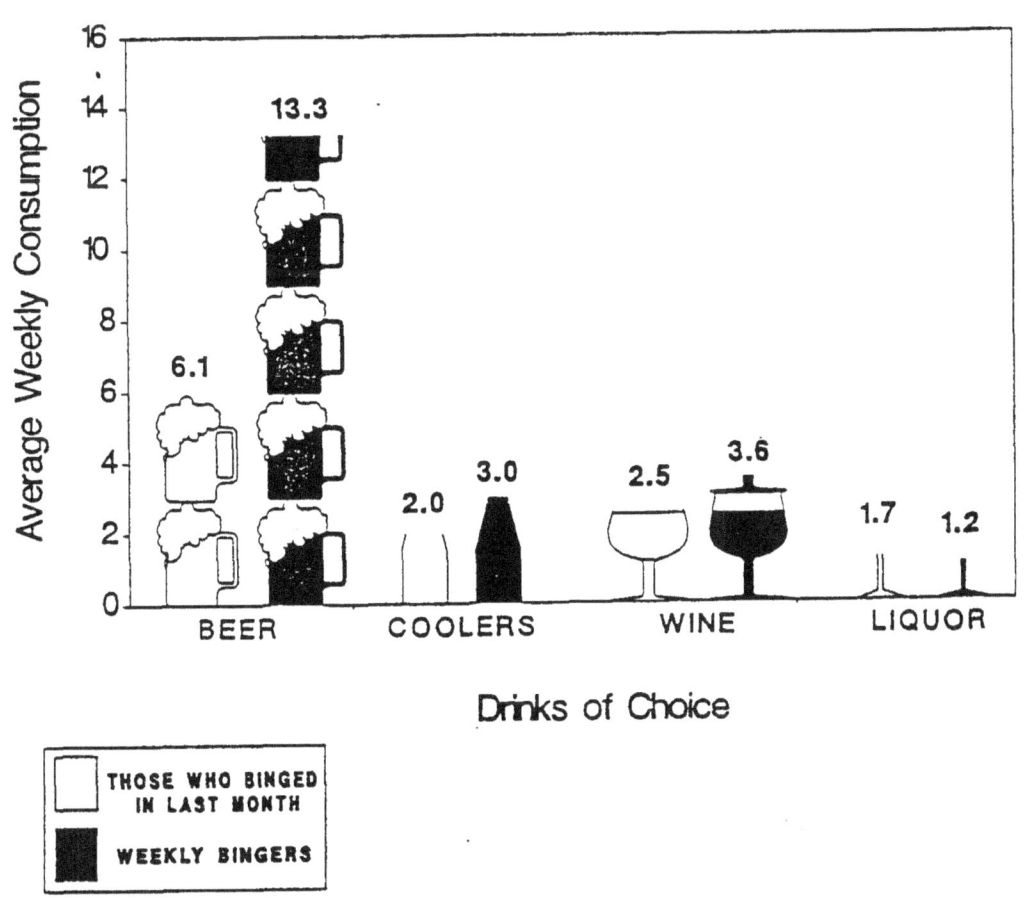

MORE THAN 3 MILLION STUDENTS DRINK ALONE, MORE THAN 4 MILLION DRINK WHEN THEY ARE UPSET, AND LESS THAN 3 MILLION DRINK BECAUSE THEY ARE BORED.

Scientific research has shown that alcohol is a fast-acting drug. The early phases of drug action tend to have a positive effect on mood and general arousal level. Many students use alcohol as a tool to help them cope with certain feelings and situations. Of the 10.6 million students who drink, (1) 31 percent drink alone, (2) 41 percent drink when they are upset because it makes them feel better, (3) 25 percent drink because they are bored, and (4) 25 percent drink to feel high.

STUDENT DRINKING PATTERNS ARE REASON FOR CONCERN

DRINKING PATTERNS

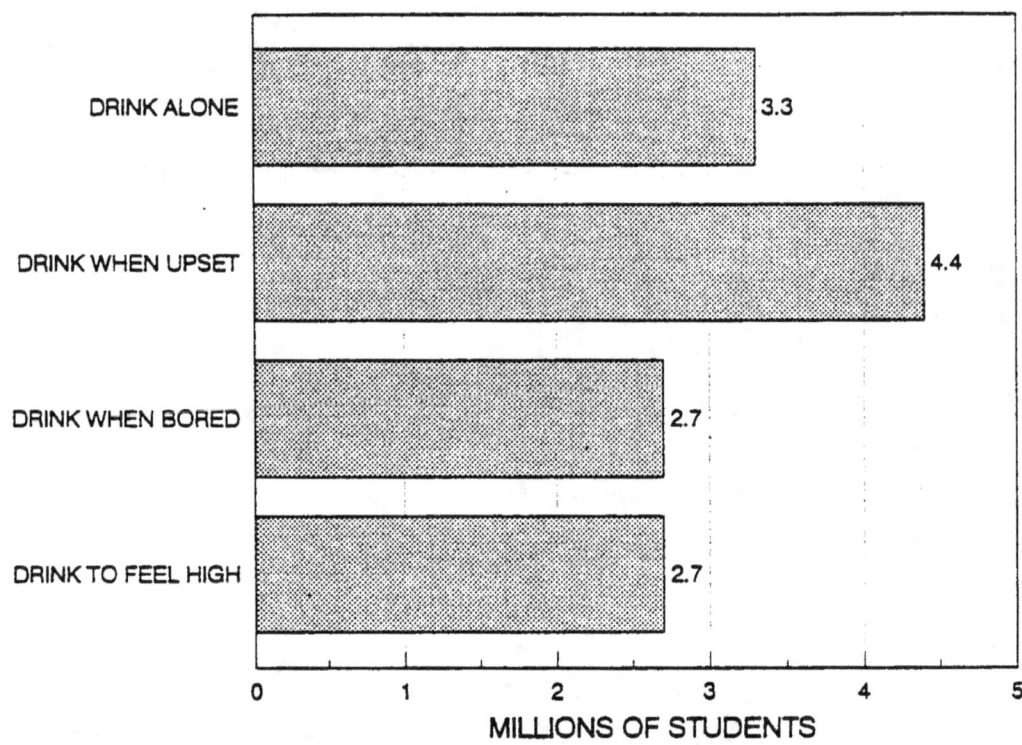

We compared these responses to a smaller group of students who binge. We found that students who binge are more likely to drink alcohol to relax, change their mood, or cope with emotional distress. Of the 5.4 million students who binge, (1) 39 percent drink alone, (2) 58 percent drink when they are upset, (3) 30 percent drink when they are bored, and (4) 37 percent drink to feel high.

STUDENTS LACK ESSENTIAL KNOWLEDGE ABOUT ALCOHOL AND ITS EFFECTS.

Nationwide, 5.6 million students are unsure of the legal age to purchase alcohol

The minimum age to purchase alcohol in all States is 21. Nevertheless, a projected 1.6 million students do not even know such a law exists. Many students know about the law, but do not know the minimum age is 21. Their guesses ranged from 14 to 24 years.

In Louisiana, only 46 percent of the students we interviewed knew the correct minimum age. The confusion among these students may be attributed to the State law which prohibits persons under 21 from purchasing, possessing, or consuming alcohol, yet does not prohibit restaurants and bars from selling alcohol to persons over 18. Therefore, someone between 18 and 21 who drinks in a restaurant has committed a violation, but the restaurant or bartender has not. A State Alcohol Beverage Commission official said they are "not prosecuting the underage drinker because the law is superficial. When servers realize this, they are not hesitant to sell to those under 21."[9]

A third of all students do not understand the intoxicating effects of alcohol

We asked students about alcohol's intoxicating effects and whether different stimulants will counteract these effects. More than 2.6 million students do not know a person can die from an overdose of alcohol. More than one-third of students believe that drinking coffee, getting some fresh air, or taking a cold shower will "sober you up."

In addition, a projected 259,000 students think that wine coolers or beer cannot get you drunk, cannot make you sick, or cannot do as much harm as other beverages. Students like wine coolers because they are "like soda--I don't consider them alcohol," and "they...don't get you drunk."

Students do not know the relative strengths of different alcoholic beverages.

Almost 80 percent of the students do not know that one shot of whiskey has the same amount of alcohol as a 12-ounce can of beer. Similarly, 55 percent do not know that a 5-ounce glass of wine and a 12-ounce can of beer have the same amount of alcohol. One out of three students do not know that all wine coolers contain alcohol.

The chart on the next page details student responses to our questions.

---

[9]May 1, 1991, telephone conversation with a State Alcohol Beverage Commission official.

ACTUAL QUESTION	CORRECT ANSWER	PERCENT CORRECT
Mothers who drink alcohol during pregnancy have a higher risk of having babies with birth defects.	True	98
Alcohol slows the activity of the brain.	True	96
A teenager cannot become an alcoholic.	False	96
Alcohol improves coordination and reflexes.	False	93
A person can die from an overdose of alcohol.	True	87
Many wine coolers actually contain no alcohol.	False	68
Drinking coffee, getting some fresh air, or taking a cold shower can help a person "sober up" more quickly.	False	54
One can of beer (12 ounces) has more alcohol than a glass of wine (5 ounces).	False	45
One shot of whiskey (1-1/2 ounces) has twice as much alcohol as a can of beer (12 ounces).	False	21

NINE MILLION STUDENTS GET THEIR INFORMATION ABOUT ALCOHOL FROM UNRELIABLE SOURCES.

More than 4 million students learn about alcohol from their friends, whose information may or may not be accurate. Similarly, more than 5 million students say that they "just picked up" what they know by themselves or that nobody taught them. A greater proportion of students who drink than non-drinkers learn about alcohol through unreliable sources. When asked who taught him about alcohol, one student explained, "Nobody. A lot of teenagers who drink it don't know what it is."

Students also learn about alcohol from their parents, school, and the media. The chart on the next page illustrates students' information sources.

STUDENTS ALSO LEARN ABOUT ALCOHOL FROM FAMILY, SCHOOL, AND THE MEDIA

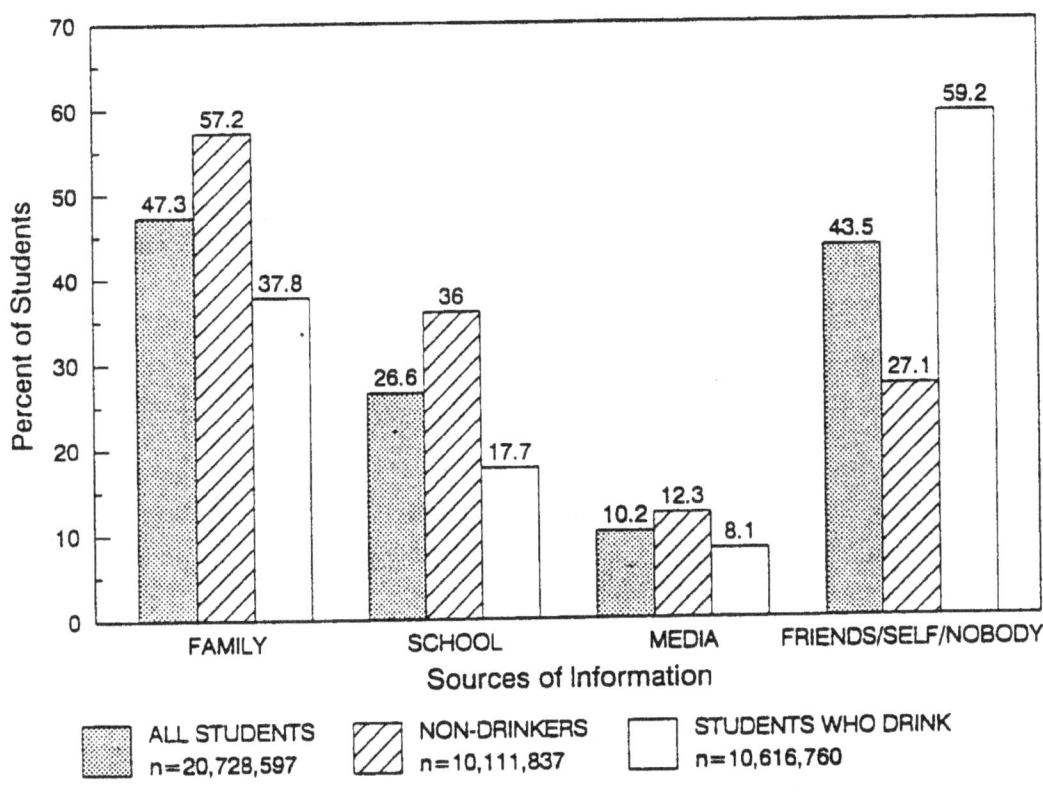

As shown in the graph, non-drinkers are much more likely to learn about alcohol from their family and school than are students who drink. Non-drinkers are also slightly more likely to cite the media as a source of their knowledge.

More than a quarter of all students cited school, a class, teachers, or a specific school program as teaching them about alcohol. For example, a few students mentioned the Drug Abuse Resistance Education (D.A.R.E.) program. A coordinated effort between local police and schools, D.A.R.E. sends uniformed police officers into the schools to teach 5th- and 6th-grade students about alcohol and other drugs.

SEVEN MILLION STUDENTS ARE ABLE TO WALK INTO A STORE AND BUY ALCOHOL.

Students can buy alcohol in stores.

Almost two-thirds or 6.9 million of the students who drink buy their own beverages. Despite the minimum age laws, students as young as 12 or 13 said they can buy alcoholic beverages in a store. As students get older, a larger proportion buy alcohol directly. Students said, "Sometimes they [vendors] do not even ask your age," and "I could go out right now and buy some."

Students may (1) use fake identification, (2) buy from stores known to sell to young people or stores with young clerks, or (3) just go in and buy alcohol. Forty-five percent of all students know someone who has used a fake identification to buy alcohol. A small group, 4.5 percent, admit they steal alcohol from stores. Unable to purchase alcohol from stores, students in Philadelphia, Pennsylvania use a black market source. Students mentioned that houses, called "speakeasies," sell alcohol to underage students, and they offer some alcoholic beverages, like Cisco, which are not available elsewhere in the State.

Friends, parties, and stores are the main sources for alcohol.

Students who drink usually obtain alcohol from their friends. Their grade in school influences where and how they get alcohol. While 88 percent of 12th graders get alcohol through friends, only 49 percent of 7th graders do. The younger students obtain alcohol from their parents with or without their parents' knowledge. Almost three-fourths of the 7th graders obtain alcohol from their parents, while only a quarter of the 12th graders do.

Almost 65 percent of all students--students who drink and non-drinkers alike--have been to parties where alcohol is served. The number of students attending parties increases with each grade level. More than 79 percent of high school students (9th through 12th grade) have been to parties with alcohol. When asked where they obtain alcohol, 88 percent of the students who drink mentioned parties.

STUDENTS ACCEPT RIDES FROM FRIENDS WHO HAVE BEEN DRINKING.

In 1989, almost 2,800 students between 15 to 19 years old died in alcohol-related traffic accidents. Forty-five percent of the traffic accidents among this age group are alcohol related, yet students say it is not okay to drink and drive.[10]

Even though 92 percent of all students in our survey said a person should never drink and drive, almost a third have accepted a ride from a driver who had been drinking. This translates to 6.8 million students who are placing their lives in danger. Almost half of the students who drink have been a passenger in a car that a friend drove after drinking.

---

[10]U.S. Department of Transportation, National Highway Traffic Safety Administration, Fatal Accident Reporting System: 1989 Annual Report, Pub. No. DOTHS807693, March 1991.

PARENTS, FRIENDS, AND ALCOHOLIC BEVERAGE ADVERTISEMENTS INFLUENCE STUDENTS' ATTITUDES ABOUT ALCOHOL

Parents influence students' attitudes about alcohol

Almost two-thirds of all students say their parents do not approve of underage drinking or would punish them if they drank. Some extreme examples of punishment that students gave are, "I would have a grave," "I would be grounded until I was 42," and "They would beat my behind!"

Many parents are more lenient. Thirty-five percent of the students who drink say their parents tolerate their drinking under certain conditions. These conditions typically limit the amount, frequency, or location of the student's drinking. Examples include, "They tell me not to go overboard and not to get drunk" and "I can have it with my parents." Almost 15 percent of the students who drink reported that their parents trust them or do not say or do anything about their drinking.

Friends influence students by providing both alcohol and occasions to drink.

Nationwide, 10.1 million students drink with their friends. The main reasons students gave for drinking involve their friends:

► Almost 8.7 million students drink to have fun.

► Less than 5.5 million students, or half of those who drink, do so because their friends drink.

► More than 6 million drink to be social.

At one of the surveyed schools, the March cover story from the student newspaper discussed student views on drinking beer. The article listed reasons why beer is so popular, including "it makes even the most shy people witty and clever at parties."[11] Some students expressed concerns that the most popular weekend activity is drinking. One student was disappointed that "several of my friends can't be social unless they are drunk (or so they say)."[12]

Advertisements for alcoholic beverages influence students' perceptions about alcohol

Thirty-nine percent of all students named something they like about advertisements for alcoholic beverages. Their likes vary widely. The most common responses were

---

[11]D. Roberts, "True Love, or Just an Alcoholic?" <u>Complex Review</u>, March 1991, p. 6.

[12]B. Linas, "Social Drinking? <u>Complex Review</u>, March 1991, p. 7.

13

that the advertisements spotlight attractive people and make drinking look like fun. We asked students if anything appealed to them about the advertisements. Student responses included:

- "They are very convincing. They make it look very glamorous."

- "The way they make life look like fun."

- "They look exciting and fun. The message is: It is all right to drink, not that it is bad."

- "Some of them are funny, and some have sexy women."

- "They make you look like you're cool and accepted."

- "Girls in the ads are skinny, and I want to be like that."

- "The slogan 'The Right Beer Now' makes you think 'Is now a good time to drink?'"

Virtually all students have seen advertisements for alcoholic beverages. To find out if students were able to associate a spokesperson, star, or symbol with a particular brand of beer, we asked the students if Spuds MacKenzie is the mascot for Coors Light beer. More than half knew that "Spuds" was not Coors' mascot. Because the majority knew enough to correctly link the symbol and the product, advertisements may be a stronger influence on students than they realize.

RECOMMENDATIONS

THE SURGEON GENERAL SHOULD CONSULT WITH PUBLIC AND PRIVATE AGENCIES TO DEVELOP, IMPROVE, AND PROMOTE EDUCATIONAL PROGRAMS WHICH WOULD INCREASE STUDENT AWARENESS OF ALCOHOLIC BEVERAGES AND THEIR EFFECTS.

This recommendation is similar to one that appears in the OIG report entitled "Youth and Alcohol: A National Survey--Do They Know What They Are Drinking?" In addition to HHS, agencies should include the U.S. Departments of Education, Transportation, and Justice, the alcohol beverage industry, and public interest groups. The Surgeon General should ensure that alcohol education is developed and improved to include practical information about alcohol. Programs should emphasize information about (1) different alcoholic beverages and their relative strengths, (2) how alcohol affects the body, (3) how to cope with problems, and (4) laws regarding youth and alcohol.

THE SURGEON GENERAL SHOULD COLLABORATE WITH THE APPROPRIATE PUBLIC AND PRIVATE AGENCIES TO REDUCE THE APPEAL OF ALCOHOLIC BEVERAGE ADVERTISING TO YOUTH.

The Surgeon General should initiate a collective effort to eliminate images that glamorize drinking or link drinking to fun, recreation, or sex appeal. We found that youth most frequently pay attention to this type of advertising which they may perceive as making drinking socially acceptable. The collective effort should include agencies such as the Bureau of Alcohol, Tobacco, and Firearms, the Federal Trade Commission, the National Association of Broadcasters, the American Association of Advertising Agencies, the alcohol industry, and public interest groups.

THE SURGEON GENERAL SHOULD EMPHASIZE THE NEED FOR LAW ENFORCEMENT AND STATE ALCOHOLIC BEVERAGE CONTROL AGENCIES TO PREVENT YOUTH FROM ILLEGALLY PURCHASING ALCOHOL.

The Surgeon General should consult the State Alcoholic Beverage Control (ABC) agencies to find ways to better deter youth from purchasing alcohol and vendors from selling to minors. The OIG will provide the Surgeon General with information about the ABC agencies and the State laws and enforcement in a subsequent report on youth and alcohol.

APPENDIX A

METHODOLOGY

Four-Stage Sampling Methodology

At the first stage, a cluster of eight States out of the nation was selected at random, without replacement, with probability proportionate to size. That is, for this level, size, defined as the number of schools in each State, was used as the weighting factor for the selection of the eight States. The universe of schools was limited to secondary schools (junior high or senior high) and Kindergarten through 12th grade schools.

The second stage involved selecting a cluster of counties within each of the eight States. Two counties were selected from each sampled State for a total of 16 counties. These counties were also selected with probability proportionate to size. However, the size for this stage was determined by the number of students in the county in grades seven through twelve.

Once counties were selected, a simple random sample of schools within the county was chosen. Two schools per county were sampled for a total of 32 schools.

The final stage of sampling was the selection of students in the schools. A sample of thirty students per school was desired. However, 42 were initially selected to allow for absentees and refusals. The schools were instructed to alphabetize a list of all students in grades 7 through 12. Then the total number of students on the list was divided by 42 and rounded to the nearest whole number (n). Students were then selected by counting every nth one on the list until the entire list was exhausted. In many cases, more than the required thirty students were available to participate. The schools were instructed to randomly subsample to obtain a final sample of 30. This final sample size was achieved in all but a few schools. However, in no school were less than 27 students interviewed. The total sample for this inspection was 956 students.

Weighting Procedure

Since the sample was selected with four different stages and a different set of probabilities at each stage, weighting of the respondents was standardized through a five-step process based on sample size and the universe. Although the first two stages of selection employed probability proportionate to size, the measure of size differed between the two stages. In the first stage the measure of size was number of schools while the measure of size for the second stage was number of students. The third and fourth stages involved taking simple random samples of schools and then students. To provide a uniform unit of selection so that accurate weights could be determined, the number of students, known at each of the four stages, was used for purposes of weighting the sample.

Overall, there were 32 distinct weights used to project to the universe--1 for each school. These weights were applied to every student in the school and were computed as follows:

(1)   In weighting from the students to the school, the population in the school was divided by the sample in the school. There were 32 different weighting factors for this phase.

(2)   The second weighting factor was determined by dividing the number of students in the county by the sum of students in the two schools that were chosen. There were 16 different weighting factors used in projecting to the county level.

(3)   In the third stage, the weight was computed by dividing the number of students in the State by the sum of students in the two counties that were chosen. There were 8 weighting factors (one for each State) at this stage.

(4)   For the final stage, the weight was calculated by taking the number of students in the universe and dividing by the number of students in all eight States combined, for one weighting factor to project to the universe.

(5)   The weight at each of these 4 stages was multiplied together to obtain the 32 unique weighting factors.

Adjustments to Weights

It was determined, subsequent to data collection, that the 956 students interviewed were disproportionately distributed when compared to the estimated national population. Using data provided by the Department of Education, we determined that the data needed to be reweighted to appropriately reflect this national population. The table on the next page shows the distribution of the national population and sample with respect to race and grade, including the adjusted weights.

DISTRIBUTION OF POPULATION AND SAMPLE
WITH RESPECT TO GRADE

GRADE	UNWEIGHTED SAMPLE	ADJUSTED WEIGHTED SAMPLE	POPULATION
7	21.40%	12.90%	13.03%
8	27.10%	12.10%	12.04%
9	14.70%	23.20%	23.32%
10	12.70%	21.40%	20.96%
11	12.40%	17.10%	17.20%
12	11.50%	13.40%	13.42%

DISTRIBUTION OF POPULATION AND SAMPLE
WITH RESPECT TO RACE

RACE	UNWEIGHTED SAMPLE	ADJUSTED WEIGHTED SAMPLE	POPULATION
WHITE	58.20%	70.20%	69.35%
BLACK	29.30%	15.40%	15.36%
HISPANIC	8.40%	10.50%	10.20%
INDIAN	0.20%	0.40%	1.04%
ASIAN	3.40%	3.40%	3.43%
OTHER	0.70%	-	-

As can be seen from the above two tables, there is a difference between the unweighted sample and population distributions with respect to both race and grade. Using a cross tabulation of race and grade, compiled for the population and the sample, the adjusted weights were constructed. These adjustments were made based on the proportions found in the sample compared with the population. For example, since whites were under sampled and blacks were over sampled, the responses were weighted more heavily for whites and less for blacks. This adjustment brought the sample in line with the national population.

The differences between the adjusted proportions and the unweighted proportions in the sample are mainly due to the following:

(1)   In general, the sample selected proportionately more 7th and 8th graders than are found in the population and,

(2)   The sample selected proportionately more non-white students than are present in the national population.

Discussion Guides

We asked all students one or two screening questions:

(1) EXCLUDING CHILDHOOD SIPS THAT YOU MIGHT HAVE HAD FROM AN OLDER PERSON'S DRINK, HAVE YOU EVER HAD A GLASS OF BEER OR WINE, A WINE COOLER, OR A DRINK OF LIQUOR?

(2) HAVE YOU HAD AT LEAST ONE DRINK IN THE PAST YEAR?

Students who answered "Yes" to both screening questions were asked questions about their personal experiences, knowledge, and attitudes about alcohol. Students who answered "No" to either of the screening questions were asked about their perceptions and observations concerning classmates who drink.

APPENDIX B

PROJECTED UNIVERSE BY GRADE AND GENDER

Our sample is representative of the 20.7 million 7th through 12th grade students in the United States. The data in this chart reflect a national projection of the students we interviewed.

GRADE	MALE		FEMALE		TOTAL	
	PERCENT	POPULATION	PERCENT	POPULATION	PERCENT	POPULATION
7TH	6.0	1,248,926	7.0	1,445,489	13.0	2,694,415
8TH	6.4	1,335,556	5.8	1,203,873	12.3	2,539,429
9TH	10.3	2,139,895	12.7	2,640,591	23.1	4,780,486
10TH	10.1	2,102,594	11.1	2,305,280	21.3	4,407,874
11TH	9.9	2,053,192	7.1	1,475,387	17.0	3,528,579
12TH	7.1	1,479,801	6.2	1,289,655	13.4	2,769,456
NOT STATED	0.0	8,358	0.0	0	0.0	8,358
TOTAL	50.0	10,368,322	50.0	10,360,275	100.0	20,728,597

APPENDIX C

SELECTED BIBLIOGRAPHY

American Council on Alcoholism, Inc., "The Most Frequently Asked Questions About Teenage Drinking and Their Answers!" June 1990.

Bachman, J.G., and L.D. Johnston, "The Monitoring the Future Project: Designs and Procedures," Occasional Paper 1, University of Michigan, Institute for Social Research, Ann Arbor, Michigan, 1978.

Chassin, L., C. Tetzloff, and M. Hershey, "Self-Image and Social-Image Factors in Adolescent Alcohol Use," Journal of Studies on Alcohol, v. 46, no. 1, 1985, pp. 39-47.

Cherry, Linda et al., "Too Young to Buy and Too Young to Sell: A Case for Raising the Age of Alcohol Sellers," Horizon Services, Inc., 1989.

City of Irvine, California, Substance Abuse Task Force, Youth Alcohol Access Project, Irvine City Council, 1990.

Coate, D., and M. Grossman, "Effects of Alcoholic Beverage Prices and Legal Drinking Ages on Youth Alcohol Use," Journal of Law and Economics, v. 31, 1988, pp. 145-171.

Linas, B., "Social Drinking?" Complex Review, March 1991, p. 7.

Males, Mike, "Youth Behavior: Subcultural Effect or Mirror of Adult Behavior," Journal of School Health, v. 60, 1990, pp. 505-508.

Malvin, J.H., and J.M. Moskowitz, "Anonymous and Identifiable Self-Reports of Adolescent Drug Attitudes, Intentions and Use," Public Opinion Quarterly, v. 47, 1983, pp. 557-566.

Mosher, James F., "The Prohibition of Youthful Drinking: A Need for Reform," Contemporary Drug Problems, v. 6, no. 3, 1987, pp. 397-436.

Moskowitz, J.M., "Alcohol and Drug Problems in Schools: Results of a National Survey of School Administrators," Journal of Studies on Alcohol, v. 49, 1988, pp. 299-305.

National Clearinghouse on Alcohol and Drug Issues (NCADI), "Alcohol and Youth," NCADI Alcohol Topics Fact Sheet, January 1987, p. 1.

National Clearinghouse on Alcohol and Drug Issues (NCADI), "Alcohol Problems and Youth," NCADI Alcohol Topics Fact Sheet, January 1985, pp. 1-2.

National Families in Action, "Wine Coolers Becoming Gateway Drug," Drug Abuse Update, no. 28, March 1989, p. 12.

1989 Data, State Reports Compiled by the Beer Institute and U.S. Department of Commerce, Bureau of Census.

Roberts, D., "True Love, or Just an Alcoholic?" Complex Review, March 1991, p. 6.

Russell, Christine, "It's Easy for Underage Men to Buy Beer in the District," Washington Post Health, March 19, 1991, p. 5.

Saffer, Henry, and M. Grossman, "Beer Taxes, the Legal Drinking Age, and Youth Motor Vehicle Fatalities," Journal of Legal Studies, v. 16, 1987, pp. 351-374.

Skager, Rodney, et al., Biennial Statewide Survey of Drug and Alcohol Use Among California Students in Grades 7, 9, and 11; Report to the Attorney General, Winter 1989-90.

U.S. Department of Health and Human Services, PHS-ADAMHA-NIAAA, Seventh Special Report to the U.S. Congress on Alcohol and Health, January 1990.

U.S. Department of Health and Human Services, PHS-ADAMHA-NIDA, "Facts about Teenagers and Drug Abuse," NIDA Capsules, no. 17, 1990.

U.S. Department of Health and Human Services, PHS-ADAMHA-NIDA, "High School Senior Drug Use: 1975-1989," NIDA Capsules, no. 23, 1990.

U.S. Department of Health and Human Services, PHS-ADAMHA-NIDA, "Highlights of National Adolescent School Health Survey: Drug and Alcohol Use," NIDA Capsules, no. 28, 1988.

U.S. Department of Health and Human Services, PHS-ADAMHA-NIDA, "Highlights of National Household Survey on Drug Abuse: Population Estimates of Lifetime and Current Drug Use, 1990," NIDA Capsules, 1990.

U.S. Department of Health and Human Services, PHS-ADAMHA-OSAP, "Alcohol Use Among Children and Adolescents," Statistical Bulletin, v. 68, no. 4, October/December 1987, pp. 2-12.

U.S. Department of Health and Human Services, PHS, Office of the Surgeon General, <u>Surgeon General's Workshop on Drunk Driving: Background Papers</u>, 1988.

U.S. Department of Transportation, National Highway Traffic Safety Administration, <u>Fatal Accident Reporting System: 1989 Annual Report</u>, Pub. No. DOTHS807693, March 1991.

University of Michigan, Institute for Social Research, "Monitoring the Future: A Continuing Study of the Lifestyles and Values of Youth," February 1990.

Washington Post, "Dramatic Findings in School Drug Survey," <u>San Francisco Chronicle</u>, February 25, 1991.

The Wine Institute, Table of Commercially Produced Wine Entering Distribution Channels in the United States, by Areas Where Produced, 1985--1989.

Wittman, Friedner D., Ph.D., J.W. Grube, and P. Shane, "Survey of Alcohol and Other Drug Experiences Among Castro Valley High School Students in 1987 and 1990," September 1, 1990.